I0116777

Fearlessly Fit at Home
Your Personal Guide to Getting Fit

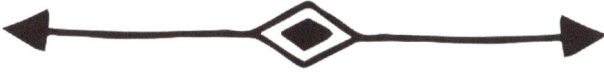

ALISA HOPE WAGNER

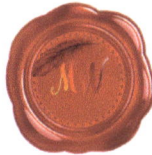

Fearlessly Fit at Home: **Your Personal Guide to Getting Fit**
Copyright @2017 by Alisa Hope Wagner
All rights reserved.
Marked Writers Publishing
www.alisahopewagner.com

Cover Design by Monica Collier
Author Photo by Lori Stead of www.wetsilver.com
Exercise photos taken by Isaac Wagner

ISBN-13: 978-0692888681 (Alisa Hope Wagner)
ISBN-10: 0692888683
BISAC: Health/Fitness/Spiritual Growth

Fearlessly Fit at Home

Your Personal Guide to Getting Fit

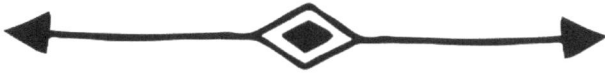

Dedication

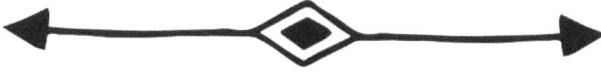

God—my Creator, Savior and Counselor

Daniel—my high school sweetheart and soul mate

Isaac—my prophet

Levi—my shepherd

Karis Ruth—my graceful companion

Christina—my awesome twin

Thank you to the women who asked if I would train them. I wrote this book for you. I might not be able to be with you in person, but I hope this book can stand in my place.

I'm so grateful to my son, Isaac Wagner, for being an amazing photographer and taking over 2,000 photos for this book. I pray many blessings in heaven for doing this for me! I'm honored that Monica Collier would take time to design a spectacular cover for this book. And, as always, thank you to Patti Coughlin for your edits and suggestions.

Introduction

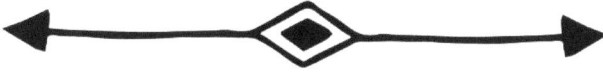

I'm a firm believer that when we begin our exercise routine, we should do it in a way that can easily be cultivated into our daily schedule. Extreme measures may work for the moment, but as they go by the wayside, so do our results. We must incorporate healthy changes that we can actually maintain, so our results are there to stay. There is nothing wrong with a kick start into fitness, but we can have our back up exercise plan ready for when life gets hectic and time and money are limited, which is why working out at home is a valid option.

This exercise program is an offshoot of my book, *Fearlessly Fit*, and it implements four necessary aspects of fitness: 1) Warm-up, 2) Cardio Calisthenics (fat burning), 3) Dumbbell Weightlifting (muscle building) and 4) Stretches. All you need for this exercise program is a towel, three sets of dumbbells (ranging from 1 pounds to 20 pounds) and motivation. Motivation can be difficult to maintain, but the benefits of having a regular workout routine will quickly materialize. You will feel and look better, and your energy will skyrocket.

We are spiritual and physical beings, and our physical health is just as important as our spiritual health. In fact, they are intertwined. We can no longer compromise our future health by skipping our daily workout routine. Because of technology (phones, cars, computers, televisions, etc.), our culture has developed a sedentary lifestyle. Therefore, working out it is not a choice, it is a requirement. We can do what it takes today to feel and look our best tomorrow. If we can do ALL things through Christ who gives us strength, we CAN achieve a healthy and fit lifestyle (Philippians 4.13).

Getting Started

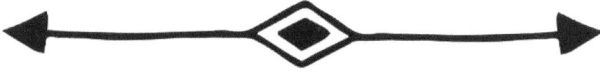

Always consult your physician or other health care professional before starting this or any other fitness program to ensure that it is right for your needs.

Purchase three sets of dumbbells, depending on your strength needs. You can choose three sets out of the following dumbbell weights: two 1-pound dumbbells, two 3-pound dumbbells, two 5-pound dumbbells, two 8-pound dumbbells, two 10-pound dumbbells, two 12-pound dumbbells, two 15-pound dumbbells or two 20-pound dumbbells.

Test each set of dumbbells, choosing the weight appropriate for working each muscle group. If you are just starting out, purchase the 1-pound dumbbells and work up from there.

If you are reluctant to buy dumbbells at the start, you can replace them with materials from your home. Milk jugs are a great way to begin a weightlifting program. You can add water to milk jugs, making them anywhere from 1 pound to 8 pounds. Save and wash two milk jugs, and they can replace the dumbbells in every exercise in this book.

This program combines both cardio and weightlifting for a full body workout that burns fat and builds muscle.

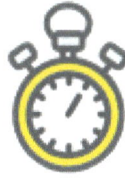

Cardio Calisthenics (CC) will increase your metabolism. Increasing your metabolism will help you burn fat, lose weight and gain energy.

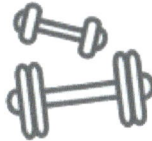

Dumbbell Weightlifting (DW) will tone and build full body muscle mass. Muscle mass is the only true fountain of youth available to you, and we want each muscle group to be strong and firm as we age.

What You Need to Know

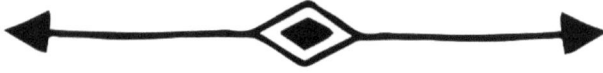

- You will boost your metabolism by performing Cardio Calisthenics. These are simple moves that spike your heart rate and work your full body, including your heart.

- Muscle mass revs up your metabolism because it takes energy to maintain it, and it will help prevent excessive muscle atrophy as you age.

- You will increase your muscle mass by performing Dumbbell Weightlifting exercises, working two muscle groups four days a week. You will target the abdominal and core one day a week.

- You will do a warm-up before your workout and stretches after. Warming up is important to prepare your body to reach its target heart rate and stretching is a necessary complement to weight training since the muscles will be tight and sore from use.

- Combining Cardio Calisthenics with Dumbbell Weightlifting is the perfect exercise combination that will give you the best results for your time.

- You will exercise five days a week for around 40-60 minutes a day at home.

- You can modify each Cardio Calisthenics exercise that calls for a jump by replacing it with a step.

- You can use the format of this program and make it your own by rearranging existing exercises, finding alternative exercises and creating new exercises. Space will be provided for you to add more exercises to this program next to each routine.

- Feel free to use the margins of this book to write down the weight you use for each of the Dumbbell Weightlifting exercises. Add the new weight next to the old as your strength increases, so you can record your progress.

The Layout

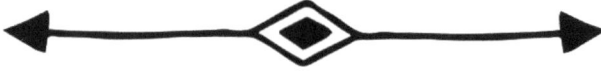

Monday:
1) Warm-up
2) Cardio Calisthenics (CC1)
3) Dumbbell Weightlifting (DW1): Quadriceps and Calves
4) Stretches

Tuesday:
1) Warm-up
2) Cardio Calisthenics (CC2)
3) Dumbbell Weightlifting (DW2): Chest and Biceps
4) Stretches

Wednesday:
1) Warm-up
2) Recovery
3) Abdominal & Core Routine
4) Stretches

Thursday:
1) Warm-up
2) Cardio Calisthenics (CC3)
3) Dumbbell Weightlifting (DW3): Hamstrings and Back
4) Stretches

Friday:
1) Warm-up
2) Cardio Calisthenics (CC4)
3) Dumbbell Weightlifting (DW4): Shoulders and Triceps
4) Stretches

Fitness Symbols

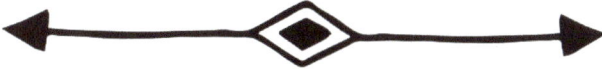

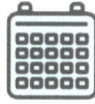

New Day

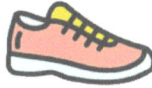

Warm up

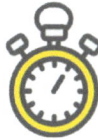

Cardio Calisthenics

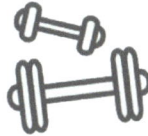

Dumbbell Weightlifting

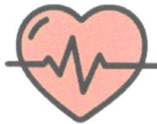

Recovery Day

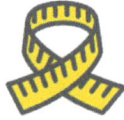

Abdominal and Core

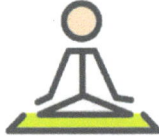

Stretches

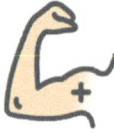

Moving On

Warm-up (5 minutes)

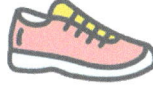

First, the warm-up increases the body temperature, warming and limbering up the muscles and connective tissues. This will increase the blood flow to all the body parts, which is necessary for the muscles to receive adequate oxygen. Next, the warm-up prepares the heart and lungs for the bulk of the workout when the target heart rate will be reached. In order to burn fat and boost the metabolism, we must ensure that we reach and maintain our target heart rate for the duration of the workout.

Finally, the warm-up transitions the mind and emotions into exercise mode, focusing all the attention on the body and exercise program. Focus is extremely important to ensuring that we implement correct form and maintain stability and balance during our workout.

Most of the warm-up moves in this program should be simple enough to perform quickly and effectively. Each exercise will be a compound move, incorporating almost every muscle in the body. With several body parts moving simultaneously, these compound exercises will increase the heart rate rapidly. Once the body is warm and the connective tissue limber, we will be less prone to injury during the more difficult portions of our workout. It is never a good idea to jump right into a rigorous cardio or weightlifting workout if the muscles and mind are not prepared.

A wonderful aspect about working out at home is that you can choose your own music to suit your mood and likes. To get ready for your warm-up and your following workout, play music that will energize and uplift you. Pick songs that have fast tempos and beats that will help you count out your reps. It is amazing what the power of music can do, so choose sounds that encourage and motivate you. Make a playlist that is at least 60 minutes long or find a radio station that plays music you love and watch just how quickly you meet your target heart rate.

You will do one set of the warm-up routine.

Warm-up exercises:
- 100 Jumping Jacks
- 100 Butt Kicks
- 100 Rope-less Jumps
- 100 Oblique Jacks
- 100 Standing Mountain Climbers

Cardio Calisthenics (15-25 minutes)

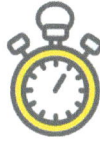

Cardio Calisthenics is a workout routine comprised of boot camp like moves that will help you hit and maintain your target heart rate for the duration of the workout. Cardio calisthenics is a full-body workout, so you will get more benefits in less time. You can do these moves from the comfort of your home because they take very little space to perform.

Each move will be counted instead of timed. Using a timer during a workout can be cumbersome, forcing your attention away from your body's form onto a clock or timer. Counting each repetition is simple, enabling you to go at your own pace and focus on each exercise. I will be providing photos of the start and finish of each Cardio Calisthenics exercise to help you correctly execute each move.

The count for the Cardio Calisthenics will be listed next to each exercise move on the exercise routine. There are five exercise moves for every set of Cardio Calisthenics. You can take a 20-count rest after each move to give you time to prepare for the next move. After each set of five Cardio Calisthenics, you can take a 60-count break before beginning the next set.

Complete each set of Cardio Calisthenics three to four times. Once you complete the third set, ask yourself if you want to go for one more set. The Cardio Calisthenics portion of your workout will take anywhere from 15 to 25 minutes. You will want to hit your target heart during your workout. Check your heart rate after each set of five Cardio Calisthenics. If you are not hitting your target heart rate, you will want to move slightly faster and take shorter breaks without compromising your form.

To check your heart rate, put the tips of your index and middle fingers on your neck just next to your windpipe, located on the carotid artery. When you feel your pulse, look at your timer (phone or watch) and count the number of beats in 10 seconds. Multiply this number by 6 to get your heart rate per minute. You want to maintain your target heart rate during the Cardio Calisthenics portion of your workout.

You will do three to four sets of the Cardio Calisthenics routine.

Age	Target HR 50-85%	Maximum HR 100%
20	100-170	200
30	95-162	190
35	93-157	185
40	90-153	180
45	88-149	175
50	85-145	170
55	83-140	165
60	80-136	160
65	78-132	155
70	75-128	150

Dumbbell Weightlifting (15-25 minutes)

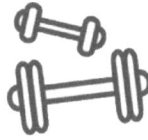

Using dumbbells is an easy way to increase muscle mass without having to go to the gym or buy expensive exercise equipment. Lifting items, like shovels, milk buckets or weaving looms were like our "dumbbell weights" centuries ago, building strength in the user's body. However, because of technological advancements today, we must replace lifting these everyday agricultural items with lifting dumbbells in order to stay healthy and strong.

We will be working two major muscle groups four days a week, including an abdominal and core workout midweek. Muscle imbalance can cause the body to become disproportionate. Our tendency to lean forward to look at the computer and phone screens is causing our back muscles to weaken and our shoulders to pull forward. We can combat this slouching phenomenon by ensuring that every muscle group, including our back, gets ample and accurate usage.

You will want to look in the mirror when you are first performing your Dumbbell Weightlifting exercises. Compare your form to the form in the photos at the start and finish of each exercise. Once you get comfortable with your form, you can begin to execute each move effectively. If you comprise your form, you may be lifting too heavy. It's best just to go down to a lighter dumbbell or simply use bodyweight. If your muscles are tight, your range of motion for each exercise may be limited. As you stretch after each workout, your body will become more limber, allowing for better range of motion.

Six major form requirements:

1) Shoulders must be rolled back. Do not slouch or roll the shoulders forward.

2) Chest must be out. This may feel awkward at first, especially if you are a woman, but keeping a proud chest is important.

3) Knees must be soft. Don't lock your knees and force your legs to be completely stiff.

4) Don't curve the back when doing low body exercises. Keep the back comfortably flat.

5) Dig the heels in the ground. Keep the toes loose enough to wiggle.

6) When picking up weights, do not bend over and pick them up. Squat, using correct form, and grab each dumbbell and lift them by using your legs, not your back.

Start out with 8 reps for each muscle group and add more as you get stronger. When performing 14 reps of an exercise becomes too easy, you will want to move up to a heavier dumbbell and go back down to 8 reps again. You will be working two muscles groups every day for around 15 to 25 minutes. Take a 20-count break in between each exercise to prepare for the next one. Once all six dumbbell weightlifting exercises are done, take a 60-count break before beginning the next set.

You will do three to four sets of the Dumbbell Weightlifting routine.

Recovery Day

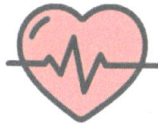

Muscle recovery is an important aspect of an exercise routine. When we do our Cardio Calisthenics and dumbbell strength training, we tear the muscle fibers in our body. "Breaking" muscle is the precursor to building it. The muscle fibers tear, and when they are adequately watered, rested and fed, they repair themselves. This process of tearing and repairing makes the muscles fibers bigger and stronger.

The midweek Recovery Day from weightlifting will allow the four muscle groups that have been worked to rest and repair themselves before working the next four muscle groups. Also, many exercises, like pushups and deadlifts, work primary and secondary muscle groups. The primary muscle group is the focus of the exercise, but the secondary muscle group is the helper. Adding a Recovery Day midweek will make sure that any secondary muscle groups that have been used are rested before working them as the primary muscle group.

Adding an Abdominal and Core routine on the Recovery Day is a great way to work on core stability, balance and strength. It will also guarantee that we will hit our target heart rate, so we can achieve our fat burning, metabolism boosting cardio for the day.

Implementing an exercise routine into our daily lifestyle will strengthen our hearts and muscles, allowing us to stay physically fit. However, exercise can cause stress on our bodies if we are not properly taking care of ourselves. When adding a workout program into our schedule, we need to check to make sure that we are preparing our bodies for the rigors of exercise. We can ask ourselves the following questions.

- Am I drinking enough **water**? Water is necessary for all the body's systems to work properly. Water flushes out waste materials that are left in the muscles after weightlifting or intense calisthenics. Always bring a large glass of water with you when you exercise.

- Am I eating enough **protein**? Without consuming enough protein, you will not be able to repair the muscle fibers that have been torn during your workout. Amino acids are the building blocks of your cells, and they are only found in protein. Eating eggs every morning is a great way to getting enough protein in your diet.

- Am I taking my **vitamins** and **minerals**? These nutrients will keep your immune system strong and are essential to all the biological processes in the body, including growing muscle. Take a multivitamin every morning to start your day.

- Am I getting enough **sleep**? Your body recovers and strengthens when it is well rested. Without enough sleep, the body will not be able to effectively accomplish a workout routine. Try to get at least 7 to 9 hours of sleep every day. Take naps when you need to catch up.

- Am I using correct **form**? Sore muscles are a normal part of a healthy exercise routine. However, strained muscles can be a sign that correct form is not being used. Practice your form in a mirror and ask a personal trainer if further instruction is needed.

Abdominal and Core (15-25 minutes)

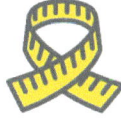

The core of the body goes from the diaphragm all the way to the pelvis, and the muscles in this area include, hip flexors, lower back, oblique and abdominal muscles. It is important to strengthen these deep muscles because they encourage the body's balance and stability, and they are the foundation for the superficial muscles of the body that we can see.

Many people make the mistake of working the superficial muscles—biceps, triceps, calf muscles and outer thigh muscles—and don't strengthen their deep core muscles. However, this will cause great muscle imbalance, which can be damaging to the body. The Abdominal and Core workout is placed in the middle of the week so all your superficial muscles can rest.

Be careful to stop if any of these core moves cause pain and check your form. If your core is weak, you will want to start carefully and slowly. Some of the listed core exercises call for a dumbbell. Use the lightest dumbbell that you have or forgo the dumbbell altogether in the beginning. As your core gets stronger, you can add the dumbbell or up the weight of your current dumbbell for more resistance.

This program has suggested reps, but you can add or take away reps depending on your needs. In addition, many of the Cardio Calisthenics and Dumbbell Weightlifting exercises throughout this program also work your core. For example, the One-legged Single Arm Rows do an excellent job at working stability. And the push-ups for chest and the single dumbbell sumo squats for the quadriceps strengthen the core. But Abdominal and Core day is a way to really target and work those deep muscles, ensuring full muscle balance.

You will do two to three sets of the abdominal core routine.

Stretches (5 minutes)

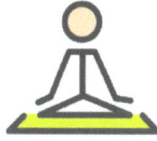

Muscles, tendons and ligaments are all sinews that can be strained while doing physical activities, which can lead to tearing of the connective tissues. The tighter these sinews are, the more prone they are to injury. When committing to an exercise program, it is imperative not to skip the stretches. Stretching is the number one way to prevent injury. Our connective tissues will not tear as easily if they are flexible.

Much of low back pain is due to tight hamstrings. We sit all day working on our computer, watching our television and driving our vehicle, so our hamstrings are in a constant stagnant position. This tightness pulls on our back muscles, causing them to ache and throb. Also, our hips are tight because we don't have many reasons to squat anymore. Tight hips can pull on our lumbar spine, compromising our posture and causing additional back pain. So much of our back pain is caused by tightness of the sinews in our body, and starting a workout program can cause additional tightness if stretching does not occur.

Grab your towel and don't skip the stretches! The stretches are performed after the workout when the muscles and connective tissues are warm and loose. Hold each stretch for 15 to 30 counts. Perform the stretch until the target area is taut and hold without breaking form. The stretch should be uncomfortable but not unbearable. If the stretch causes pain, stop immediately and check your form. It is better to ease into the stretch than to force the body to flex beyond its capacity. You can repeat the stretches in order to get a deeper stretch.

Our bodies have been shaped to fit our phones, computers, cars and televisions and correcting our posture will take time. We can enjoy our stretches more by meditating. We can meditate on how good our workout has made us feel. We can meditate on how fit our body is getting and how healthy and strong we are becoming. We can also meditate on God and His promises found in the Bible. Taking your Bible onto your towel with you while you stretch is a great way to have your quiet time with God every day. You can enjoy a devotional, read a few verses, listen to a sermon or podcast while stretching. These are all good ways to stretch your spirit as well as your body.

You will do one to two sets of the stretches routine.

Stretches:
- Hamstring Stretch (15-30 count each leg)
- Butterfly Stretch (15-30 count)
- Twisted Glute Stretch (15-30 count each leg)
- Behind Back Chest Stretch (15-30 count)
- Triceps Stretch (15-30 Count each arm)
- Plank Calf Stretch (15-30 count each leg)
- Runners Stretch (15-30 count each leg)
- Quadriceps Stretch (15-30 count each leg)

Moving On

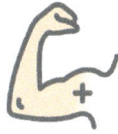

This *Personal Guide to Getting Fit* is just the beginning. There are hundreds of Cardio Calisthenics and Dumbbell Weightlifting exercises that get the heart pumping and work each muscle group. Once you become familiar with the ones listed in this program, you can start adding more moves to your repertoire of fitness knowledge. The body is an amazing machine, and it can grow accustomed to certain Cardio Calisthenics that are repeated daily. This means that the body's strength and stamina has improved, so other exercise moves are required to push the body harder. It is simple to create new lists of Cardio Calisthenics to add to this program and to switch up the ones that are listed.

Also, almost every Dumbbell Weightlifting move listed in this program can be slightly altered to activate the muscles in different ways. Any Google search on a certain weightlifting move will offer several different modifications to the exercise. There are usually images and videos that will help you achieve and keep good form. Further, you will want to make sure that you are increasing your resistance little by little. Once a certain weightlifting exercise is accurately performed with the most number of reps, it is time to move up in weight. You can slowly purchase more dumbbells and add them to your growing home gym.

Lastly, dumbbells are just the beginning! Adding exercise equipment to your home gym over time is an awesome investment to your health—body, mind and soul. Physical activity is linked to greater mental alertness, better moods, sounder sleep, less fatigue, decreased depression and a heightened sense of wellbeing. The body releases chemicals called endorphins that give the body a natural, healthy high, which triggers positive feelings. Feeling good every day is just another important reason to make exercise an integral lifestyle choice. When you add equipment to your home gym little by little, you can become more creative and diverse with your workout routine. Add new exercises to this routine as you increase your fitness knowledge in the spaces provided.

Suggested additional exercise equipment:

1) Exercise mat. A mat offers the body more cushion while doing floor exercises.

2) Exercise gloves. Gloves will protect your hands from getting blisters and give them more support while doing Dumbbell Weightlifting.

3) Exercise bench. This will allow you to perform lying down weightlifting moves off the floor, enlarging your range of motion.

4) Bar and plate weights. You can achieve a greater amount of weightlifting moves when using a bar. Plus, plate weights can be used alone for many exercises.

5) Bosu ball. Doing weightlifting moves or Cardio Calisthenics on a Bosu ball can add greater stability and balance to your workout routine.

6) Kettlebells. These can be used instead of dumbbells for certain moves where a better grip is needed.

7) Medicine ball. You can replace the dumbbell with the medicine ball and add a variety of new Cardio Calisthenics and abdominal and core exercises to your workout program.

Monday

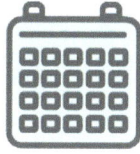

I. **Warm-up:** One set
1) 100 Jumping Jacks
2) 100 Butt Kicks
3) 100 Rope-less Jumps
4) 100 Oblique Jacks
5) 100 Standing Mountain Climbers
6) _____
7) _____
8) _____

II. **CC1:** Three to four sets
1) Power Skips (40 reps)
2) Jumping Lunges (10 reps each side for 20 total)
3) High Knees (20 reps each leg for 40 total)
4) Bell Jumps (10 reps front and back for 20 total)
5) Crab Kicks (20 reps each side for 40 total)
6) _____
7) _____
8) _____

III. **DW1:** Three to four sets

Quadriceps:
1) Single Dumbbell Sumo Squats (8-14 reps)
2) Dumbbell Split Squats (8-14 reps each leg)

29

3) Dumbbell Squats (8-14 reps)
4) _____
5) _____
6) _____
7) _____

Calves:

1) Calf Raises with Dumbbells (8-14 reps)
2) Pigeon Calf Raises with Dumbbells (8-14 reps)
3) Plié Calf Raises with Dumbbell (8-14 reps)
4) _____
5) _____
6) _____
7) _____

IV. **Stretches:** One to two sets

1) Hamstring Stretch (15-30 count each leg)
2) Butterfly Stretch (15-30 count)
3) Twisting Glute Stretch (15-30 count each leg)
4) Behind Back Chest Stretch (15-30 count)
5) Triceps Stretch (15-30 Count each leg)
6) Plank Calf Stretch (15-30 count each leg)
7) Runners Stretch (15-30 count each leg)
8) Quadriceps Stretch (15-30 count each leg)
9) _____
10) _____
11) _____
12) _____

Tuesday

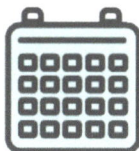

I.   👟 **Warm-up:** One set
1) 100 Jumping Jacks
2) 100 Butt Kicks
3) 100 Rope-less Jumps
4) 100 Oblique Jacks
5) 100 Standing Mountain Climbers
6) _____
7) _____
8) _____

II.   ⏱ **CC2:** Three to four sets
1) 180 Jump Squats (10 reps each side for 20 total)
2) Squat Punches (30 reps each side for 60 total)
3) Vertical Jumps (20 reps)
4) Hopscotch Jumps (20 reps)
5) Plank Salutes (20 reps each side for 40 total)
6) _____
7) _____
8) _____

III.   🏋 **DW2:** Three to four sets

Chest:
1) Push-ups (8-14 reps)
2) Lying down Dumbbell Chest Presses (8-14 reps)

3) Lying Down Chest Flies (8-14 reps)
4) _____
5) _____
6) _____
7) _____

Biceps:
1) Hammer Curls (8-14 reps)
2) Bent Over Single Concentration Curls (8-14 reps each arm)
3) Standing Inner Bicep Curls (8-14 reps)
4) _____
5) _____
6) _____
7) _____

IV.   **Stretches:** One to two sets
1) Hamstring Stretch (15-30 count each leg)
2) Butterfly Stretch (15-30 count)
3) Twisting Glute Stretch (15-30 count each leg)
4) Behind Back Chest Stretch (15-30 count)
5) Triceps Stretch (15-30 Count each leg)
6) Plank Calf Stretch (15-30 count each leg)
7) Runners Stretch (15-30 count each leg)
8) Quadriceps Stretch (15-30 count each leg)
9) _____
10) _____
11) _____
12) _____

Wednesday

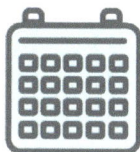

I. **Warm-up:** One set
1) 100 Jumping Jacks
2) 100 Butt Kicks
3) 100 Rope-less Jumps
4) 100 Oblique Jacks
5) 100 Standing Mountain Climbers
6) _____
7) _____
8) _____

II. **Recovery Day:** Allow the muscle groups to rest

III. **Abdominal & Core Routine:** Two to three sets

Lying Down:
1) Russian Twists (20 reps each side for 40 total)
2) Overhead Crunch Rotations (10 reps each side for 20 total)
3) Bicycle Abdominals (20 reps each side for 40 total)
4) Abdominal Flutter Kicks (20 reps each leg for 40 total)
5) Vertical Leg Crunches (20 reps)
6) _____
7) _____
8) _____

Standing:
1) Dumbbell Twists (10 reps each side for 20 total)
2) Dumbbell Oblique Raises (20 reps each side for 40 total)
3) Dumbbell Wood Chops (10 reps each side for 20 total)
4) Dumbbell Single Knee Raises (10 reps each side for 20 total)
5) Dumbbell Overhead Side Bends (10 reps each side for 20 total)
6) _____
7) _____
8) _____

IV. **Stretches**: One to two sets
1) Hamstring Stretch (15-30 count each leg)
2) Butterfly Stretch (15-30 count)
3) Twisting Glute Stretch (15-30 count each leg)
4) Behind Back Chest Stretch (15-30 count)
5) Triceps Stretch (15-30 Count each leg)
6) Plank Calf Stretch (15-30 count each leg)
7) Runners Stretch (15-30 count each leg)
8) Quadriceps Stretch (15-30 count each leg)
9) _____
10) _____
11) _____
12) _____

Thursday

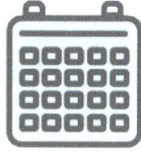

I. **Warm-up:** One set
1) 100 Jumping Jacks
2) 100 Butt Kicks
3) 100 Rope-less Jumps
4) 100 Oblique Jacks
5) 100 Standing Mountain Climbers
6) _____
7) _____
8) _____

II. **CC3:** Three to four sets
1) Burpee Jumps (10 reps)
2) Single Leg Swings (10 reps each leg for 20 total)
3) Frog Jumps (10 reps back and forth for 20 total)
4) 180 Lunges (10 reps each side for 20 total)
5) Plank Toe Side Touches (10 reps each side for 20 total)
6) _____
7) _____
8) _____

III. **DW3:** Three to four sets

Hamstrings:
1) Good Mornings (8-14 reps)

2) Dumbbell Romanian Deadlifts (8-14 reps)
3) Hamstring Dumbbell Bridges (8-14 reps each leg)
4) _____
5) _____
6) _____
7) _____

Back:
1) Bent Over Dumbbell Rows (8-14 reps)
2) One-legged Single Arm Rows (8-14 reps)
3) Bent Over Dumbbell Reverse Flies (8-14 reps)
4) _____
5) _____
6) _____
7) _____

IV. **Stretches:** One to two sets
1) Hamstring Stretch (15-30 count each leg)
2) Butterfly Stretch (15-30 count)
3) Twisting Glute Stretch (15-30 count each leg)
4) Behind Back Chest Stretch (15-30 count)
5) Triceps Stretch (15-30 Count each leg)
6) Plank Calf Stretch (15-30 count each leg)
7) Runners Stretch (15-30 count each leg)
8) Quadriceps Stretch (15-30 count each leg)
9) _____
10) _____
11) _____
12) _____

Friday

I. Warm-up: One set

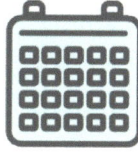

1) 100 Jumping Jacks
2) 100 Butt Kicks
3) 100 Rope-less Jumps
4) 100 Oblique Jacks
5) 100 Standing Mountain Climbers
6) _____
7) _____
8) _____

II. CC4: Three to four sets

1) Side to Side Single Leg Hops (20 reps each side for 40 count total)
2) Standing Knee Crunches (20 reps each leg for 40 total)
3) Ski Jumps (10 reps each side for 20 total)
4) Crossover Punches (40 reps)
5) Floor Mountain Climbers (10 reps each leg for 20 total)
6) _____
7) _____
8) _____

III. DW4: Three to four sets

Shoulders:
1) Standing Dumbbell Presses (8-14 reps)
2) Dumbbell Front Raises (8-14 reps each arm)
3) Bent Over Dumbbell Flies (8-14 reps)
4) _____
5) _____
6) _____
7) _____

Triceps:
1) Lying Down Dumbbell Skull Crushers (8-14 reps)
2) Standing Overhead Dumbbell Triceps Extensions (8-14 reps)
3) Bent Over Kickbacks (8-14 reps)
4) _____
5) _____
6) _____
7) _____

IV.   **Stretches:** One to two sets
1) Hamstring Stretch (15-30 count each leg)
2) Butterfly Stretch (15-30 count)
3) Twisting Glute Stretch (15-30 count each leg)
4) Behind Back Chest Stretch (15-30 count)
5) Triceps Stretch (15-30 Count each leg)
6) Plank Calf Stretch (15-30 count each leg)
7) Runners Stretch (15-30 count each leg)
8) Quadriceps Stretch (15-30 count each leg)
9) _____
10) _____
11) _____
12) _____

Exercise Photo Guide

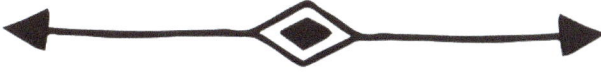

Warm-up

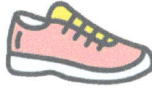

Jumping Jacks

Start with feet together, knees soft and arms at the side. Jump moving legs more than shoulder width apart and bringing the arms overhead. Jump back to starting position.

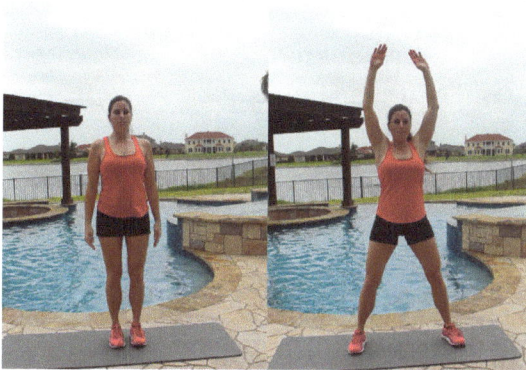

Butt Kicks

Keeping the torso erect, jog in place while trying to kick the heels as close to the glutes as possible.

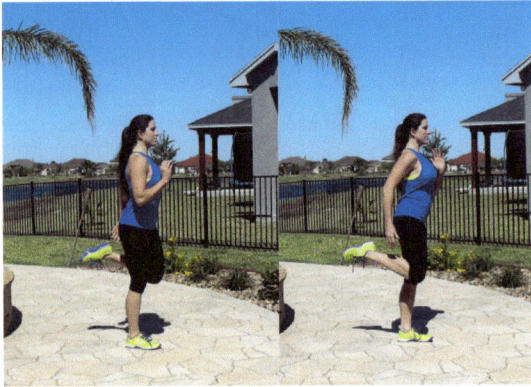

Rope-less Jumps

Stand with feet hip width apart, torso erect and hands holding the ends to an imaginary rope out to the side. Jump with both feet simultaneously while turning the wrists.

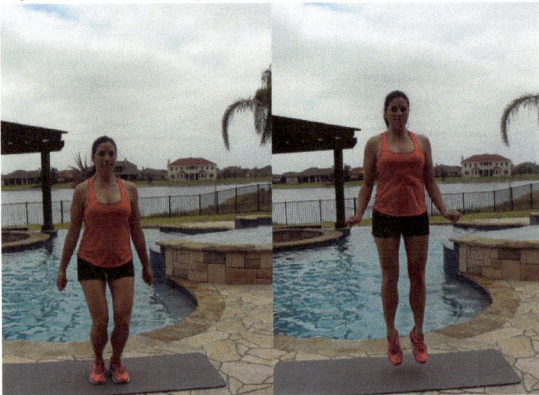

Oblique Jacks

Stand with feet hip width apart and place your hands behind your head. Jump while bending your right knee up and leaning your right elbow toward your knee, bending your torso to the right. Then jump again and do the same move on the left side.

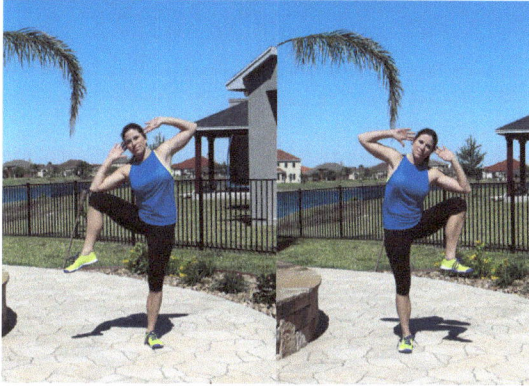

Standing Mountain Climbers

Hop from the left foot to the right foot, bringing the knees up toward the torso while raising the opposite hand to the ceiling. Try to only have one foot on the floor at a time.

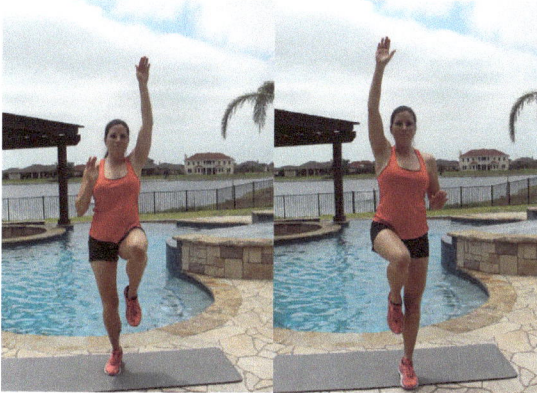

Monday: CC1

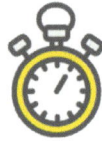

Power Skips
Stand with core tight and feet hip width apart. Lifting the right knee, spring up from the left foot while stretching the left arm toward the ceiling. Repeat on the opposite side.

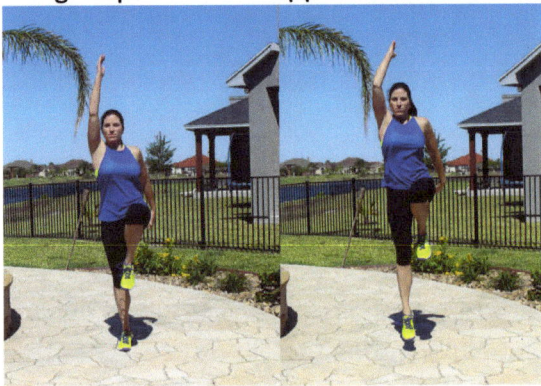

Jumping Lunges
Stagger legs in a lunge and jump off both feet, keeping your core tight and knees soft. Land with the opposite leg in front at a 90-degree angle and back leg bent. Jump back to starting lunge.

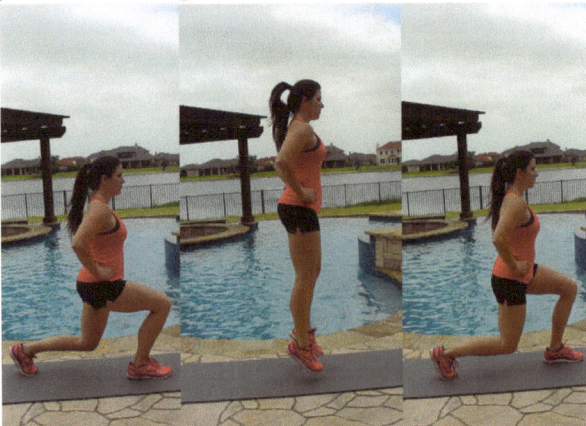

High Knees

Keeping torso erect, jog in place while bringing the knees up toward the hips. Land softly.

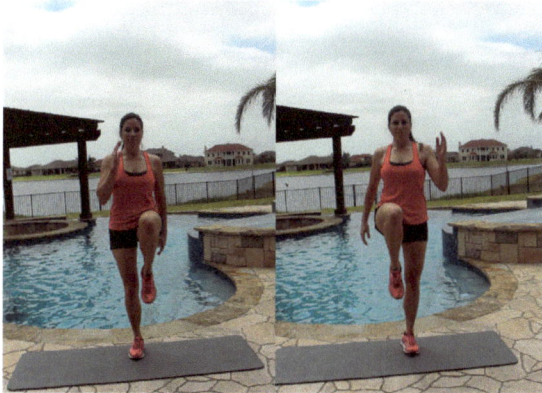

Bell Jumps

Stand with legs hip width apart, keeping knees slightly bent and core tight. Jump from both feet and land 1-2 feet in front of you. Then jump back to starting position, landing softly.

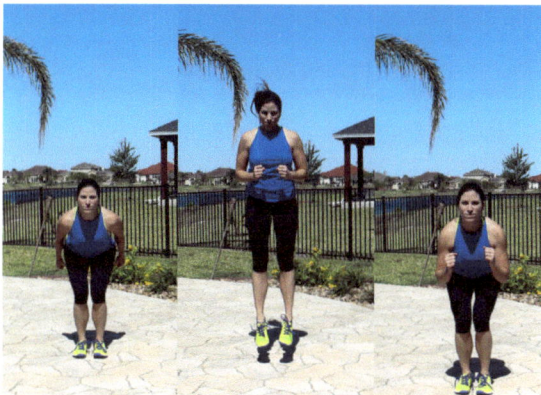

Crab Kicks

Sit down with legs in front of you, knees bent and feet together. Place your palms to the ground behind you with your fingers facing back. Lifting your hips off the ground, kick your right leg up. Then kick the left leg up as the right leg descends back to the ground.

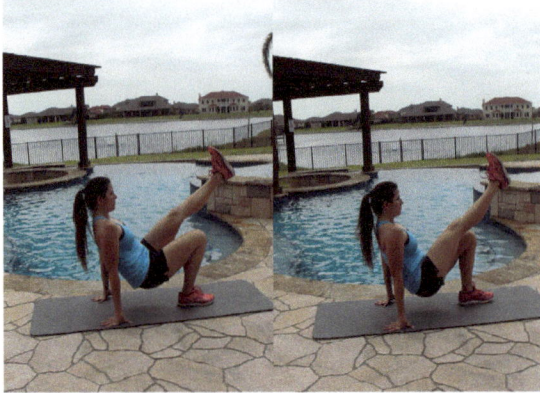

Monday: DW1

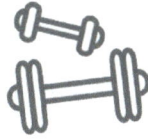

Quadriceps

Single Dumbbell Sumo Squats

Stand with legs more than shoulder width apart with toes pointing out. Keep core tight and shoulders back, holding single dumbbell between the legs. Bend knees into squat, keeping back flat. Return to starting position.

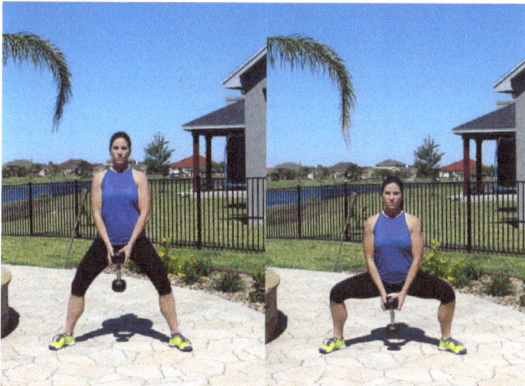

Dumbbell Split Squats

Stand with feet together, chest out and knees soft. Step one foot in front of you, making a 90-degree angle. Return leg and alternate feet. Keep back flat and back foot stationary.

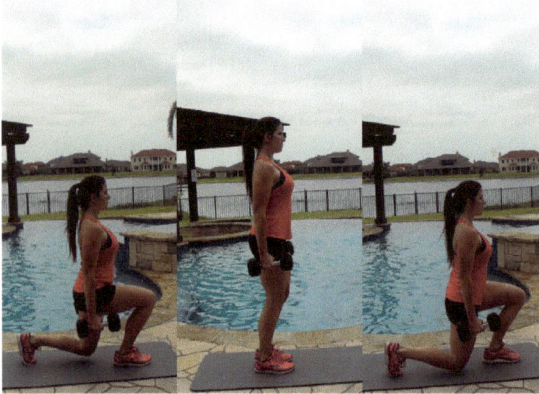

Dumbbell Squats

Stand with legs shoulder width apart, torso erect, shoulders back and knees soft. Hold a dumbbell in each hand with the arms at the side and palms facing in. Push your glutes back and bend the knees into a squat position, keeping the back flat. Then dig in your heels, pushing the body back up and keeping the chin lifted.

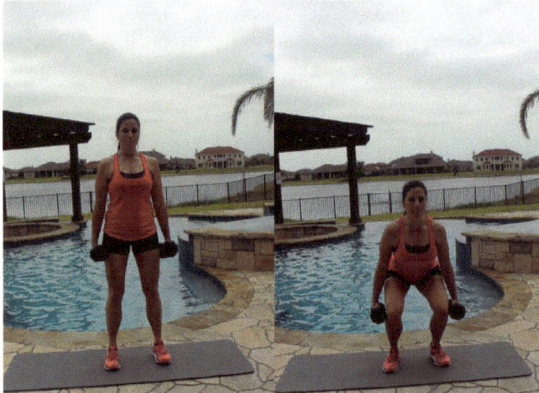

Calves

Calf Raises with Dumbbells

Hold dumbbells on either side of the body with palms facing in. Feet should be a little less than shoulder width apart. Keep your torso erect and shoulders back and lift onto your toes.

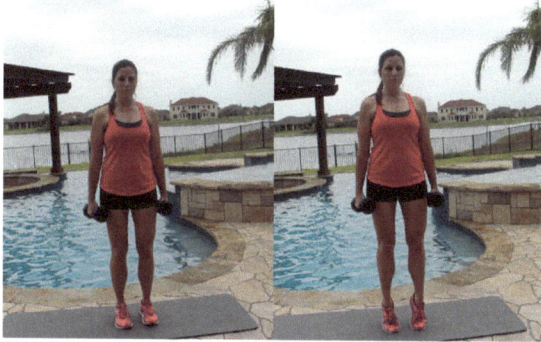

Pigeon Calf Raises with Dumbbells

Hold dumbbells on either side of the body with palms facing in. Place toes close together and heals out. Keep your torso erect and shoulders back and lift onto your toes.

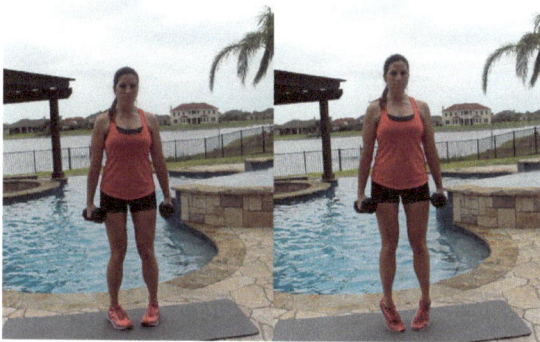

Plié Calf Raises with Dumbbell

Hold dumbbell between the legs. Place feet more than shoulder width apart and point toes out. Keep torso erect and shoulders back and lift onto your toes.

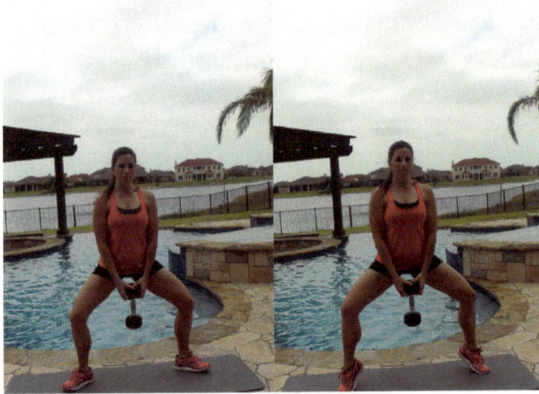

Tuesday: CC2

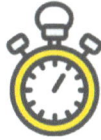

180 Jump Squats

Stand with legs hip width apart, knees soft and core tight. Facing one direction, do a deep squat. Then twist torso and jump to face the opposite direction, landing softly and keeping the back flat.

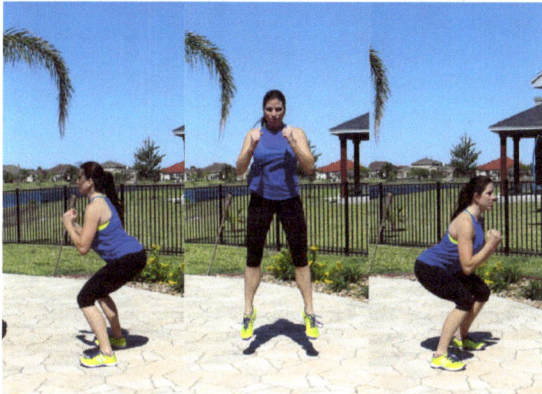

Squat Punches

Place feet hip with apart and toes pointing out. Bend knees into static squat position, keeping core tight and shoulders back. Punch left and right arm forward at eye level.

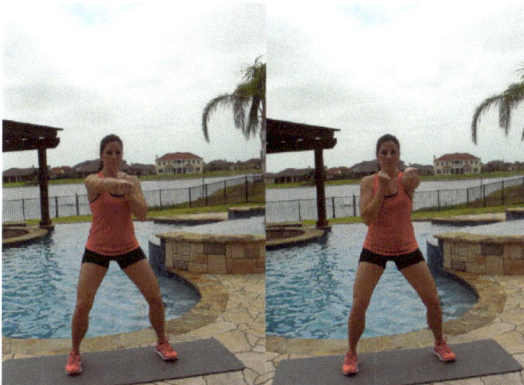

Vertical Jumps

Standing with feet hip width apart and core tight, slightly bend the knees and spring straight up with arms raising toward the ceiling. Land softly with knees slightly bent.

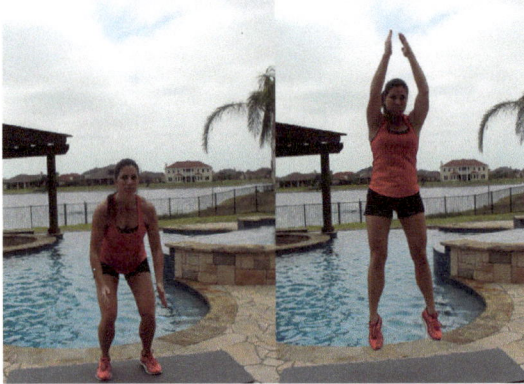

Hop Scotch Jumps

Stand with feet no more than hip width apart, knees soft and core tight. Jump forward, spreading the feet to more than shoulder width apart. Jump back to starting point with feet close together again.

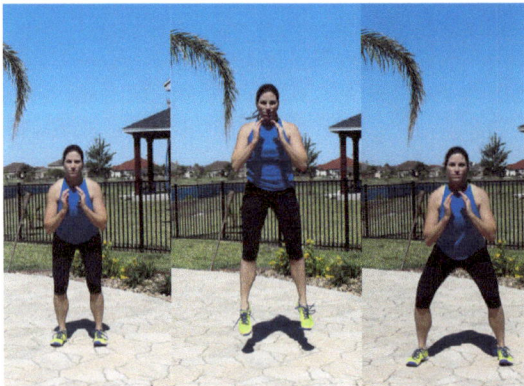

Plank Salutes

Get into plank position on the floor, resting on your palms and the balls of your feet. Bring the right arm out and forward into a salute that is aligned with the forehead. Repeat with left arm, keeping core tight.

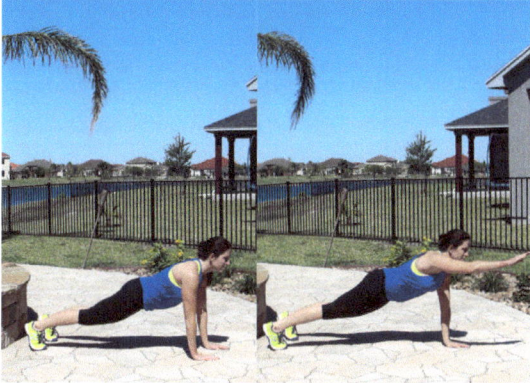

Tuesday: DW2

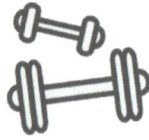

Chest

Push-ups on Toes

Put your palms on the floor a little more than shoulder width apart and fingertips facing up. Get onto the balls of the feet or the knees, keeping back flat and body parallel to the floor. Bend the elbows and bring chest just above the floor. Do not let back sag or arch. Return to starting position.

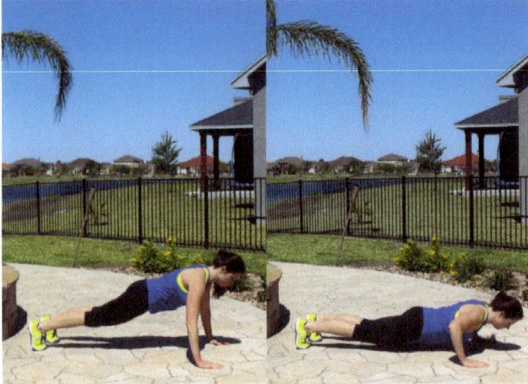

Push-ups on Knees

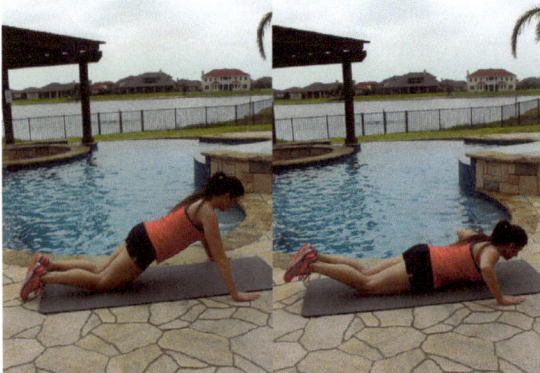

Lying Down Dumbbell Chest Presses

Lie with back on the ground, knees bent and feet planted just under the torso. Have a dumbbell horizontally in each hand with arms raised above the face and palms facing away from the body. Slowly bend the elbows, bringing the dumbbells to either side of the shoulders in a 90-degree angle. Squeeze your chest to bring the dumbbells back to starting position.

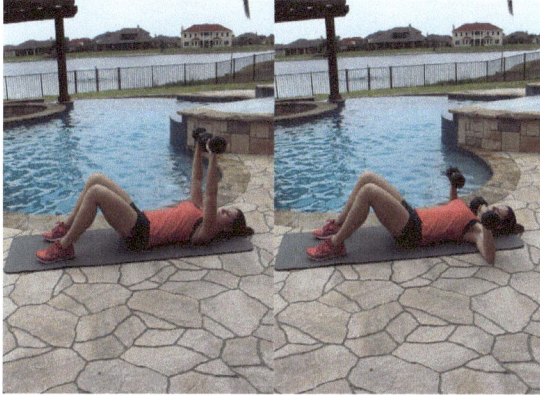

Lying Down Chest Flies

Lie with back on the ground, knees bent and feet planted just under the torso. Have a dumbbell vertically in each hand with arms raised above the chin and palms facing each other. Keep a slight curve in the arms like holding a big beach ball. Slowly widen the arms into a large arc and then bring the palms back to starting position.

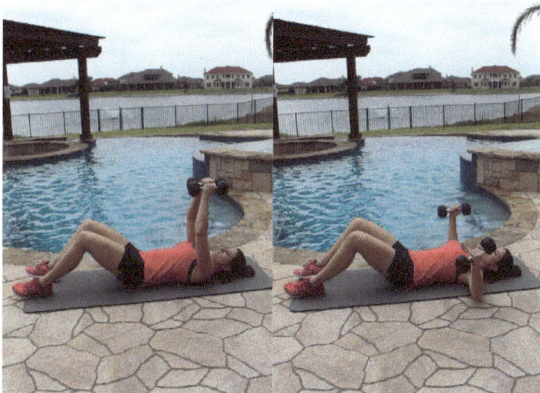

Biceps

Hammer Curls

Stand with torso erect, feet hip width apart and knees soft. Hold a dumbbell vertically in each hand with palms facing in toward the thighs. Keeping your upper arms firm, lift the dumbbells until they are shoulder level. Once biceps are completely contracted, slowly bring hands back down to hip level.

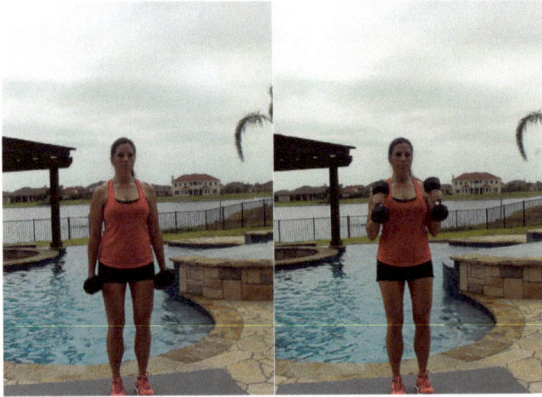

Bent Over Concentration Curls

Keep the core tight, feet shoulder width apart, toes pointing out and knees soft. Bending over, place left hand on left knee and have a single dumbbell horizontally in the right hand with palm facing out, dangling the dumbbell between the legs. Rest right elbow on inner thigh for support and bring the dumbbell towards chest in a bicep curl. Once the bicep is fully contracted, slowly bring the dumbbell down between the legs.

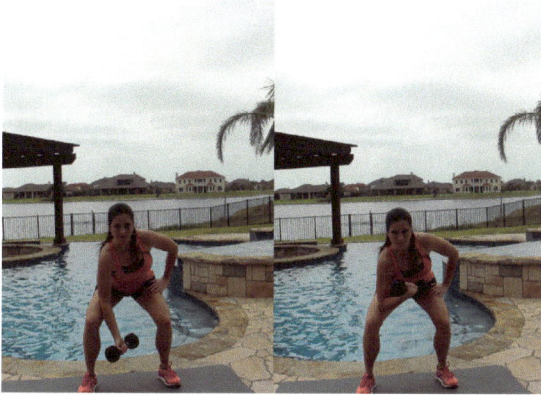

Standing Inner Bicep Curls

Stand with feet hip width apart, knees soft, torso erect and shoulders back. Place a dumbbell horizontally in each hand and let the arms dangle at each side with palms facing out. Bring the hands up in a wide curl, raising the dumbbells towards each shoulder. Once the biceps are fully contracted, slowly bring dumbbells back towards the outer thighs.

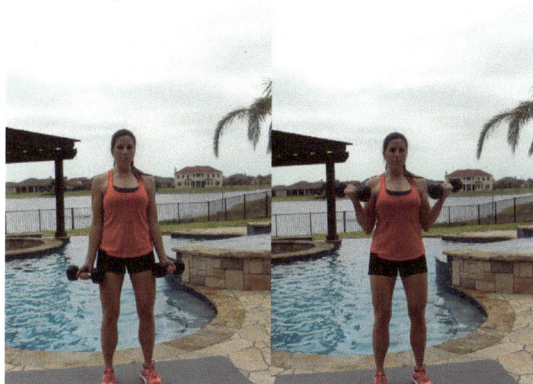

Wednesday: Abdominal and Core Routine

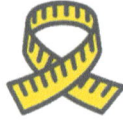

Lying Down

Russian Twists
Sit on the ground, slightly bend the knees and place your feet at shoulder width in front of you. Keeping core tight and back straight, lean your back toward the floor until your abs contract. Stretch your arms and claps your hands in front of you. Slowly twist from the right side to the left side, pausing for 2 counts at each side.

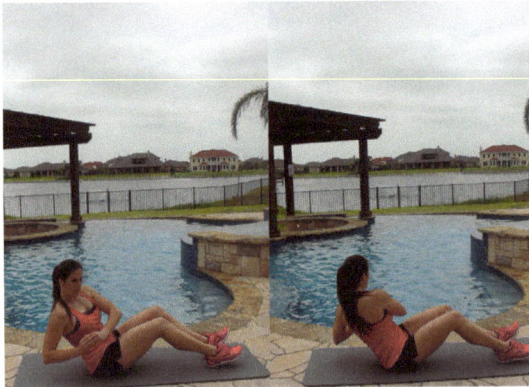

Overhead Crunch Rotations

Lie back on the ground with knees slightly bent and feet at shoulder width in front of you. Bring arms above the head, resting on the ground and hands clasped. Keeping the core tight, lift the torso and arms up until back is almost vertical. Arms should be straight out and eye level. Then rotate torso to the left, bringing clasps hands toward the left hip. Return to starting position and repeat on the right side.

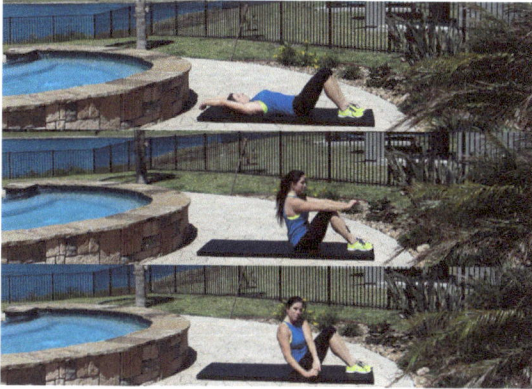

Bicycle Abdominals

Lie back on the ground with legs long and hands tucked under the head, bending at the elbows. Keeping the core tight and the feet flexed, lift the upper back a few inches off the ground and bring the right elbow to the left knee, twisting the torso and bending the left leg. Return the foot and elbow back to starting position and repeat on the other side, bringing the left elbow to the right knee.

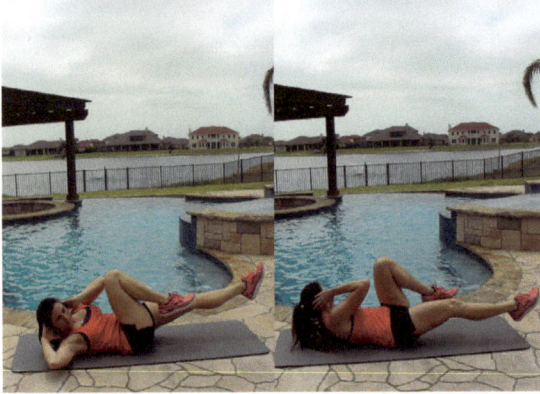

Abdominal Flutter Kicks

Lie on your back with arms resting at the side and palms facing down tucked under your lower back and glutes. Lift your feet and shoulders simultaneously several inches off the ground, activating your lower abs. Kick feet up and down in short movements just above the ground in opposite directions.

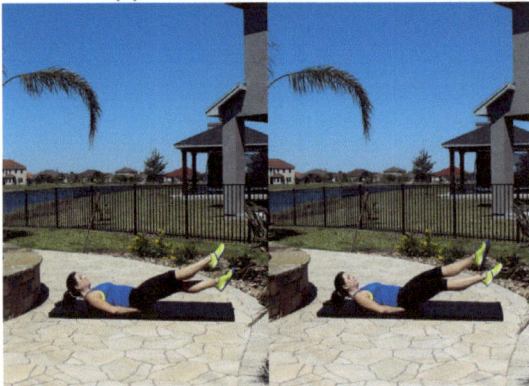

Vertical Leg Crunches

Lying flat on the ground, flex the feet and bring them up towards the ceiling above the hips. Place hands behind the head, keeping the back flat on the ground. Keeping the core tight and activating the abs, lift the shoulders into a crunch.

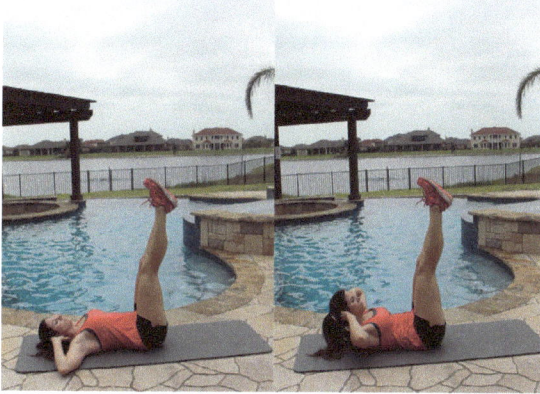

Standing

Dumbbell Twists

Stand with feet shoulder width apart and knees soft. Grasp single dumbbell with both hands, straighten arms to eye level. Keeping the core tight and shoulders back, rotate torso to the left side and bring it back to center. Then rotate the torso to the right side, bringing it back to center.

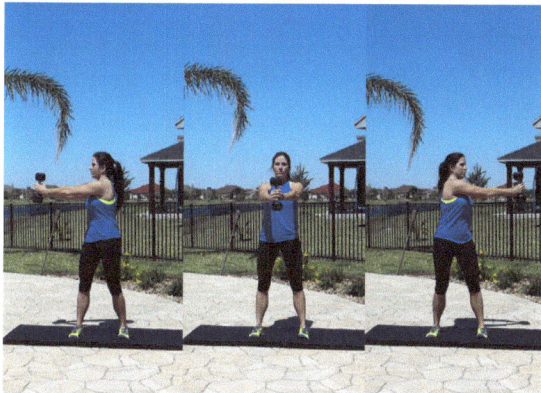

Dumbbell Oblique Raises

Stand with feet shoulder width apart and knees soft. Place dumbbell in left hand with palm facing in, dangling the dumbbell by the left side. Rest right hand on the right hip. Keeping core tight and shoulders back, bend at the waist allowing the dumbbell to move further down the left side of the body. Return to starting position and repeat on the right side.

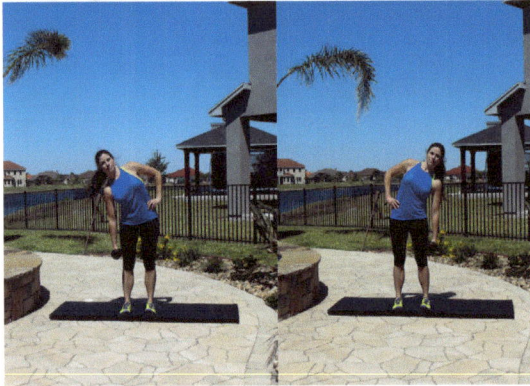

Dumbbell Wood Chops

Stand with feet shoulder width apart, holding a dumbbell with both hands above the right shoulder with your arms straight. Keep core tight and knees soft. Bring the dumbbell down across the body toward the left hip toward the left thigh. Finish reps before switching sides.

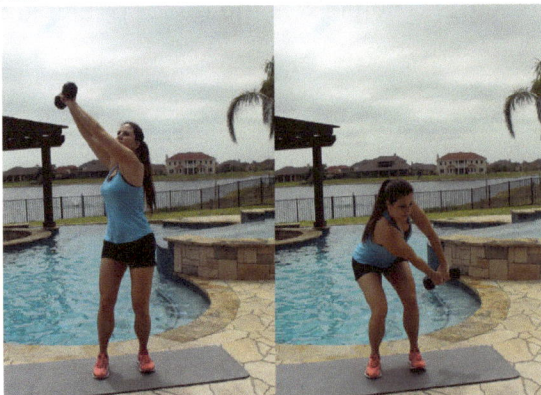

Dumbbell Overhead Side Bends

Standing with feet shoulders width apart, torso erect and knees soft, grip a single dumbbell over head with both hands. Bend at the waist to the right side, keeping the core tight and arms straight. Return to starting position and then bend at the waist to the left side.

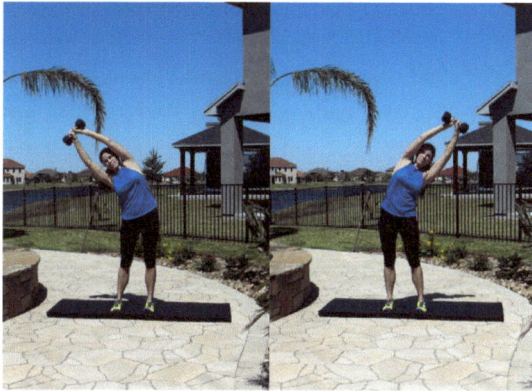

Dumbbell Single Knee Raises

Stand with feet shoulder width apart, torso erect and knees soft. Place a single dumbbell on the right thigh just above the knee. Activating the core, bend the right leg and use your abs and hip flexors to lift the knee toward your hips. Firmly hold the dumbbell horizontally in place with the right hand, placing your left hand on your hip. Then slowly bring the leg back to standing position. Finish reps before switch legs.

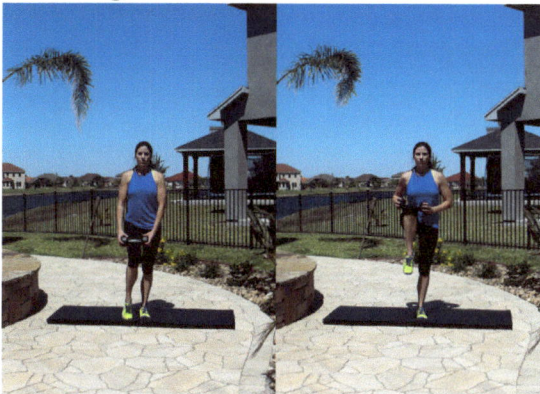

Thursday: CC3

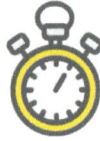

Burpee Jumps

Stand with feet shoulder width apart and knees soft. Bend the knees and hips to bring the palms flat on the ground several inches above the feet. Shoot the legs back behind you, landing on the balls of your feet in push-up or plank position. Then bring the feet back toward the palms and push up through the legs, straightening the knees. Using both feet simultaneously, jump up with arms stretched toward the ceiling and land softly.

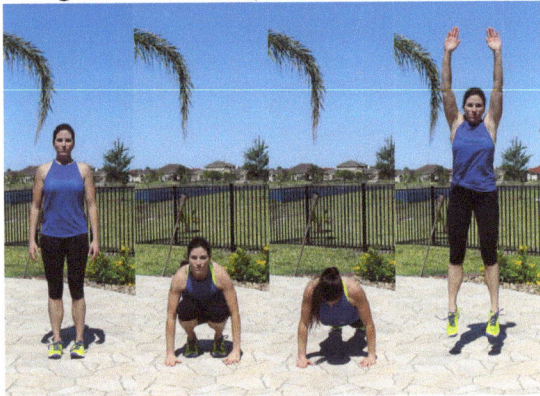

Single Leg Swings

Place feet hip width apart, keeping knees soft and torso erect. Place both hands on the hips and swing the right leg front to back, trying to get the leg parallel to the floor. Finish reps on the right side before switching to the left side.

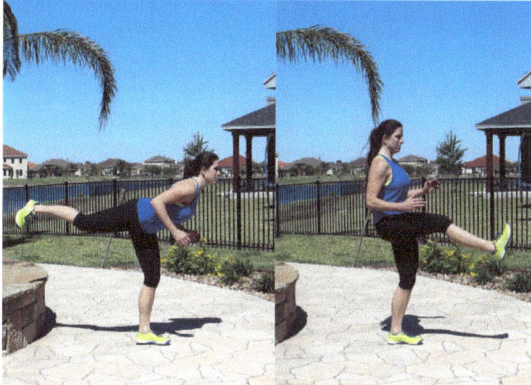

Frog Jumps

With feet shoulder width apart and knees soft, squat down and place your hands on the floor in front of your feet. Spring up from both feet, reaching your hands towards the ceiling and jumping one or two feet in front of you. Squat back down again before springing back up from both feet back to your starting position.

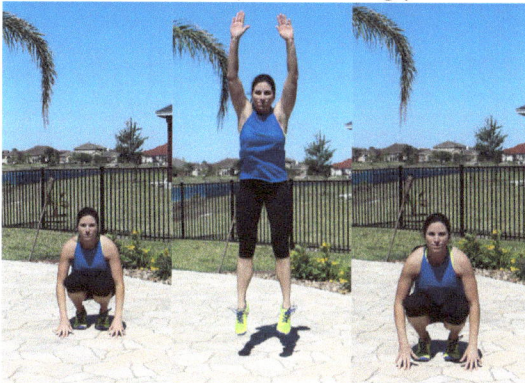

180 Lunges

Stand with feet staggered in lunge position, keeping knees soft and core tight. Facing one direction, do a deep lunge. Then twist torso and jump to face the opposite direction. Land softly with feet staggered in lunge position, facing the other side. Repeat the deep lunge before jumping back to starting position.

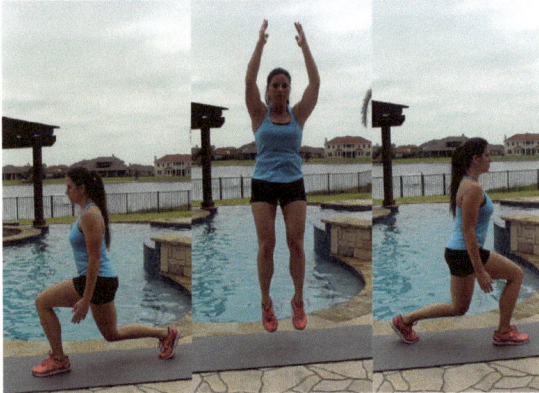

Plank Toe Side Touches

Get into plank position on the elbows and balls of the feet with body completely parallel to the floor. Move left leg out several inches and touch the toes to the ground, returning the foot back to starting position. Then move the right leg out and touch the toes to the ground.

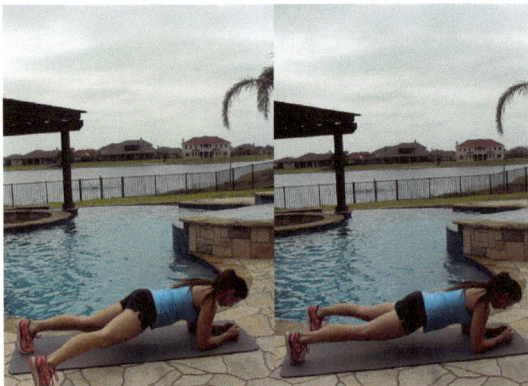

Thursday: DW3

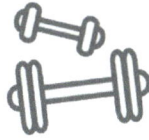

Hamstrings

Good Mornings

Stand with legs wider than shoulder width apart and toes pointing out, digging in the heals. Bring dumbbell horizontally to the chest just under the clavicle, holding the dumbbell in place with both hands. Push the glutes back and bend at the hips, bringing the torso parallel to the ground. Keep shoulders back and core tight. Hold for 2 counts and return to starting position.

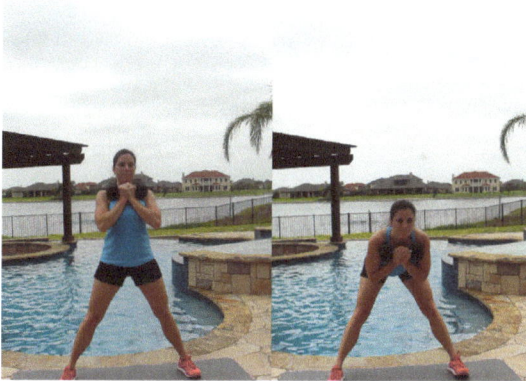

Dumbbell Romanian Deadlifts

Stand with feet hip width apart, shoulders back and torso erect. Hold dumbbells in front of you with palms facing your body. Bending at the hips, slowly push your glutes back and bend knees slightly. Keep back flat, chest out and chin up. Pause 2 counts when tension in the hamstrings stops further movement and then dig in the heals and return to starting position.

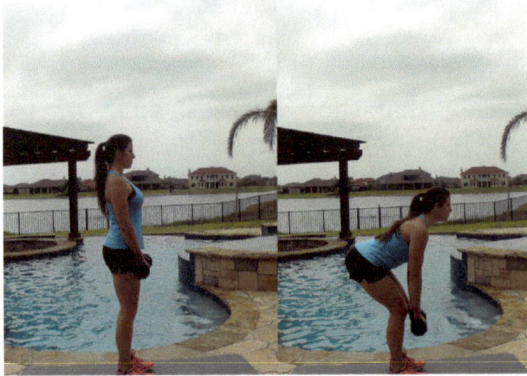

Hamstring Dumbbell Bridges

Lay flat on your back with knees bent and feet located just below the torso. Lay dumbbell horizontally across the hips, holding it in place with your hands. Bring the left leg up toward the ceiling and squeeze hamstrings and glutes, bringing your glutes off the ground. Finish reps and switch legs.

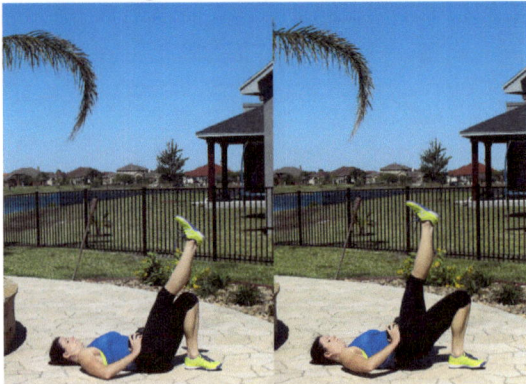

Back

Bent Over Dumbbell Rows
Stand with legs shoulder width apart, knees soft and shoulders back. Hold dumbbells in each hand with palms facing the body. Bending at the hips, bend forward and keep your back flat and core tight. Try to parallel your chest to the floor. Hanging the dumbbells directly below you, lift your elbows towards the ceiling. Keep your elbows close to the body and squeeze the back muscles.

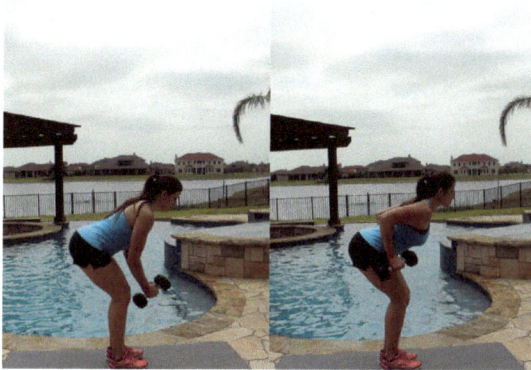

Bent Over Dumbbell Reverse Flies

Stand with legs shoulder width apart and knees soft. Hold dumbbells vertically in each hand with palms facing the body. Bending at the hips, lean forward and keep your back flat and core tight. Keep a slight curve in the arms like holding a big beach ball. Slowly widen the arms into a large arc and bring them back, squeezing the shoulder blades together.

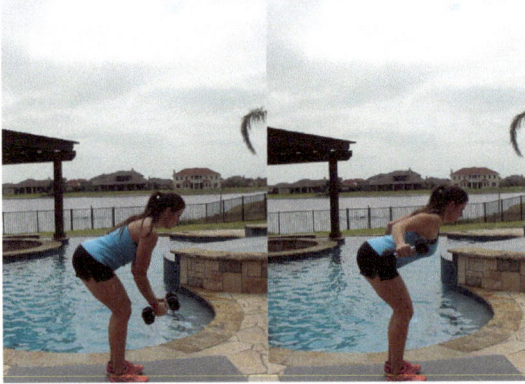

One-legged Single Arm Rows

Get on your hands and knees, keeping back flat and core tight. Hold dumbbell in the right hand with palm facing the body and keep the left palm on the ground. You can lift the left leg to add more stability training. Activate the back muscles to bring arm to 90-degrees and squeeze the shoulder blade. Finish reps and change the dumbbell to the left hand and lift the right leg.

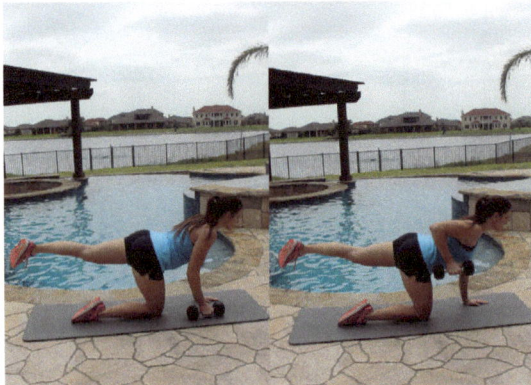

Friday: CC4

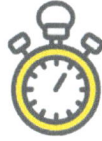

Side to Side Single Leg Hops

Standing with feet hip width apart and knees soft, hop to the right and land on the right foot. Then hop to the left, landing on the left foot. Try to hop one foot in the air and two feet from left to right, like you are hopping over a large rock.

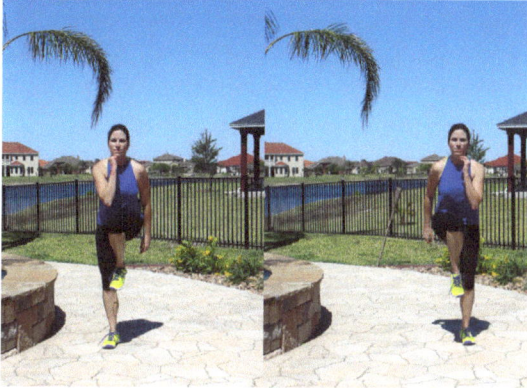

Standing Knee Crunches

Stand with feet hip width apart and core tight. Place fisted hands at shoulder level in front of you. Bring hands down to either side of the hips while raising the right knee to standing crunch position. Return to starting position and then bring left knee to standing crunch position.

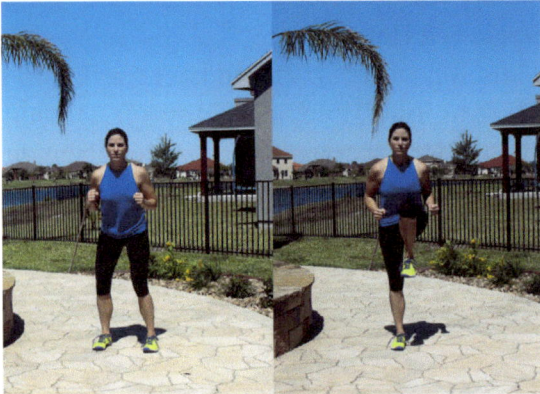

Ski Jumps

Jump side to side with feet together, springing from balls of the feet simultaneously. Bring one arm in a sweeping motion across the body in the direction of your jump.

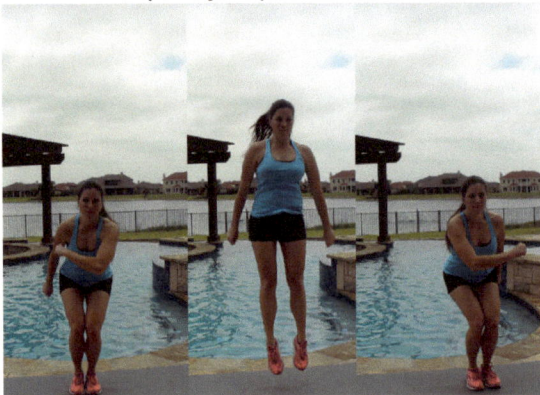

Crossover Punches

Stand with feet hip width apart and knees soft. Make hands into fist and move the right hand left across the body. Slightly turn the feet and body toward the left to follow the punch. Come back to starting position and move the left hand right across the body, moving the feet and body right to follow the punch.

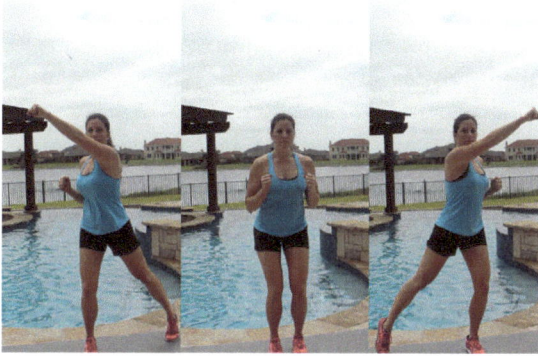

Floor Mountain Climbers

Get into plank position on the palms and balls of the feet. Keeping torso tight and body parallel to the floor, bend the left knee and bring it toward the hips. Return the left leg to starting position and bend the right knee, bringing it toward the hips. Try to transfer legs at the same time, so only one foot is on the ground at one time.

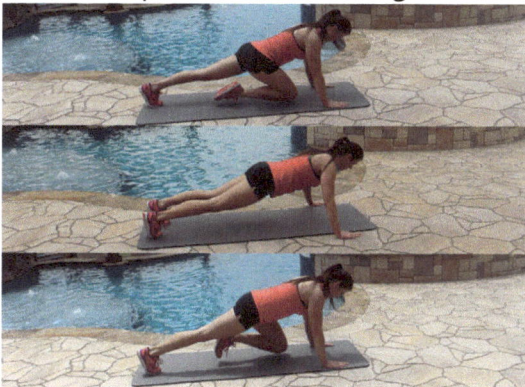

Friday: DW4

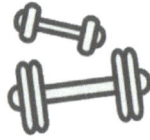

Shoulders

Standing Dumbbell Presses

Stand with feet hip width apart, torso erect and knees soft. Hold a dumbbell in each hand horizontally and bring them up to shoulder level at a 90-degree angle with palms facing out. Extend the arm through the elbows, raising the dumbbells directly above the head. Slowly return dumbbells to starting position.

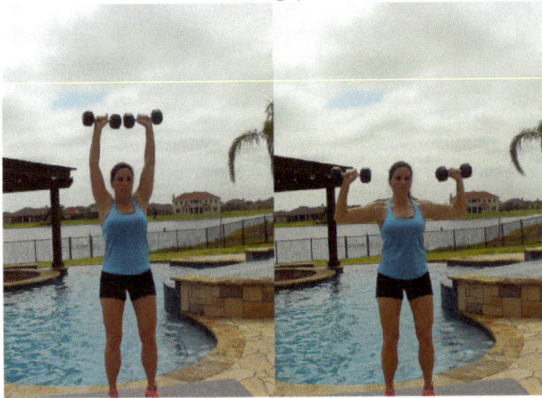

Dumbbell Front Raises

Stand with feet hip width apart, torso erect and knees soft. Hold dumbbells in each hand horizontally, palms facing the body and dumbbells resting against the thighs. Lift the right dumbbell to eye level, activating the shoulders and extending the arm. Slowly return arm to starting position and then lift the left dumbbell to eye level.

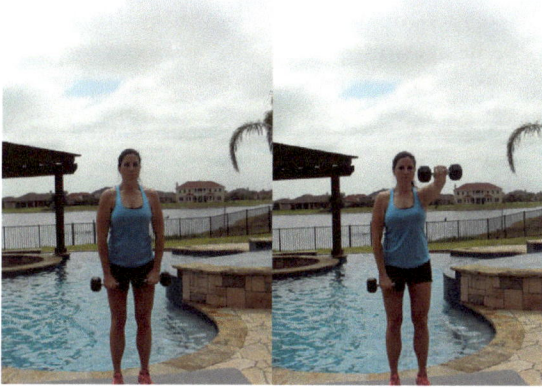

Bent Over Dumbbell Flies

Stand with legs shoulder width apart and knees soft. Hold dumbbells vertically in each hand with palms facing the body. Bending at the hips, lean forward and keep your back flat and core tight. Keep a slight curve in the arms like holding a big beach ball. Activating the shoulders, slowly widen the arms into a large arc and bring them up and out.

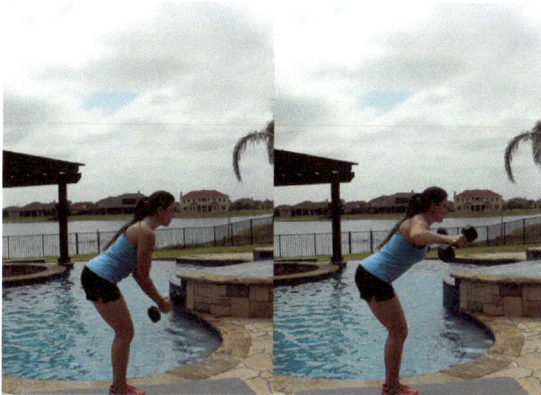

Triceps

Lying Down Dumbbell Skull Crushers
Lie down with your back to the ground, knees bent and feet placed just under the hips. Hold a dumbbell horizontally in both hands over your head with palms facing together. Bring the arms back to a 90-degree angle toward your forehead, bending from the elbows and keeping upper arms stationary.

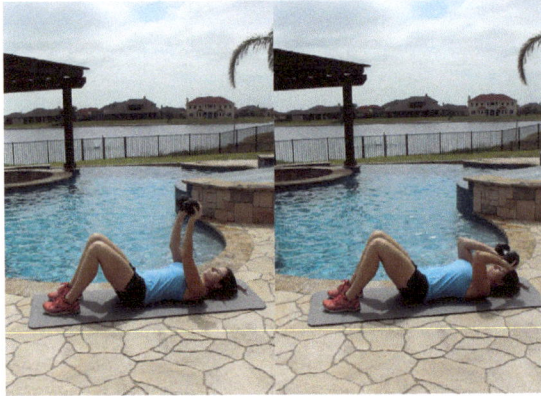

Standing Overhead Dumbbell Triceps Extensions
Stand with feet hip width apart, torso erect and knees soft. Hold a single dumbbell vertically with both hands, extending your arms over your head. The upper arms are stationary while the elbows bend, bringing the dumbbell behind the head. Prevent the elbows from going wide. Raise the dumbbell back overhead, squeezing the triceps.

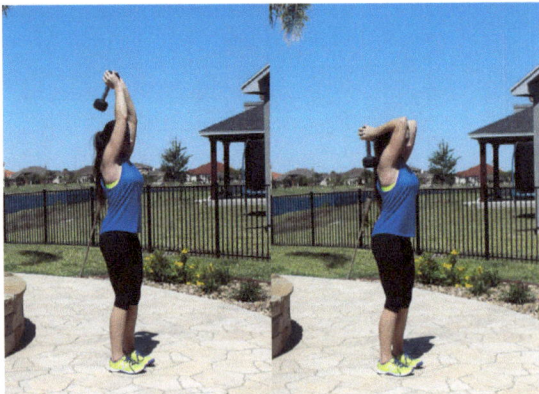

Bent Over Kickbacks

Stand with legs shoulder width apart and knees soft. Bending at the hips, lean forward and keep your back flat and core tight. Try to parallel your chest to the floor. Bring elbows to a 90-degree angle, keeping your upper arms close to the torso and stationary. Squeeze the triceps and extend the arms back. Keep your chin up and slowly return arms to the starting position.

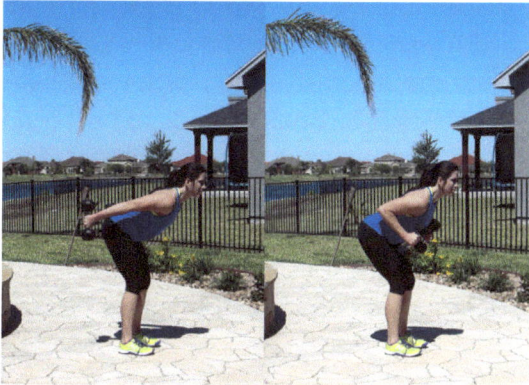

Stretches

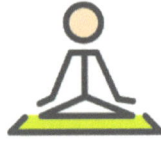

Hamstring Stretch

Sit on the floor with legs separated and knees straight. Reach hands toward the left foot, holding the stretch when the hamstring is taut. You can grasp the knee, shin, ankle or foot to help hold the stretch without bending the knee. Switch to the right foot.

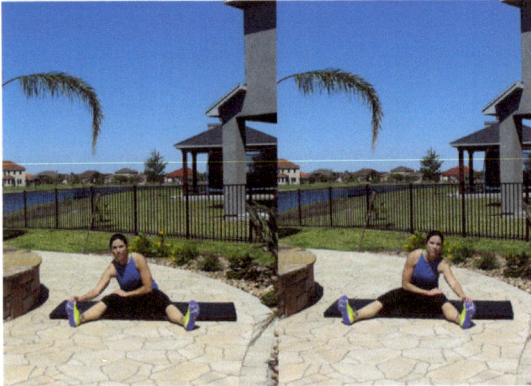

Butterfly Stretch

Sit with feet together in front of you and pulled toward your pelvis, grasping your feet with your hands. Lean your chest forward, keeping your back flat. Use your elbows to push gently on the inner thighs. The inner thigh, groin and hips should be stretched but not in pain.

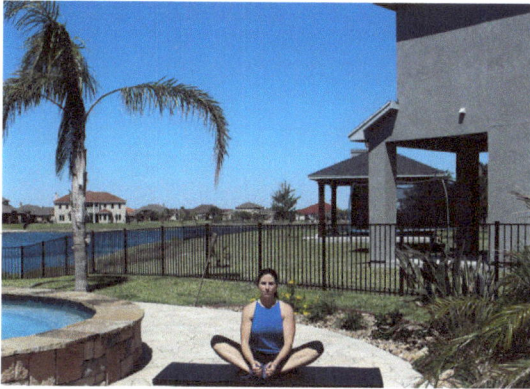

Twisting Glute Stretch

Sit on the floor with torso erect and both legs extended. Then bend the right knee, bringing the leg over the left knee or hip. Twist the torso toward the right, resting the left elbow across the bent knee. Hold the stretch and switch sides.

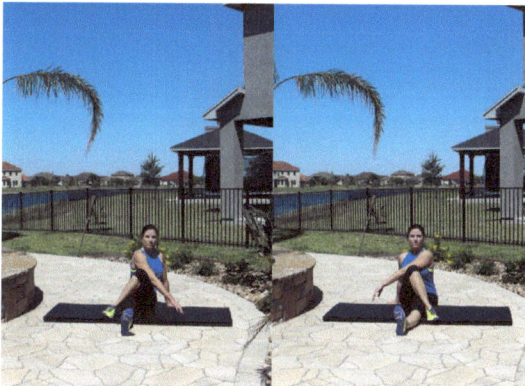

Behind Back Chest Stretch

Stand with feet hit width apart and knees soft. Reach both arms behind the back and clasp the hands together. Straighten your arms and pull your shoulder blades together and push your chest out while trying to raise the hands higher behind the back. Keep chin up.

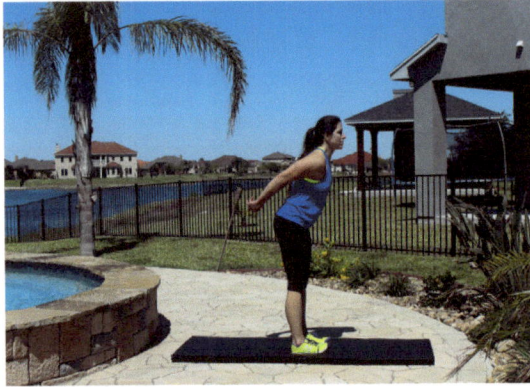

Triceps Stretch

Stand with feet hip width apart and knees soft. Lift your right arm overhead and bend the elbow, bringing your right hand toward your back with palm facing down. Use your left hand to push back on the right elbow, providing a stretch through the triceps. Switch arms.

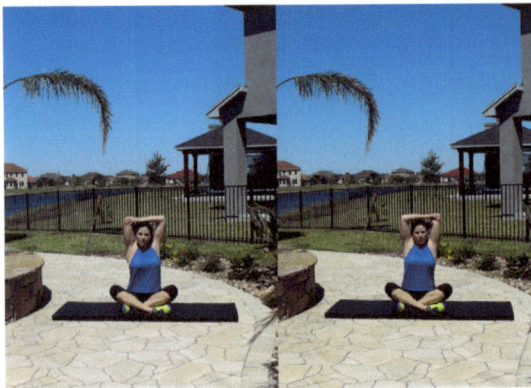

Plank Calf Stretch

Get in plank position on palms and balls of the feet. Push your glutes up and back, making a "V" shape with your body and stretch the calves by pushing each heal toward the floor one at a time.

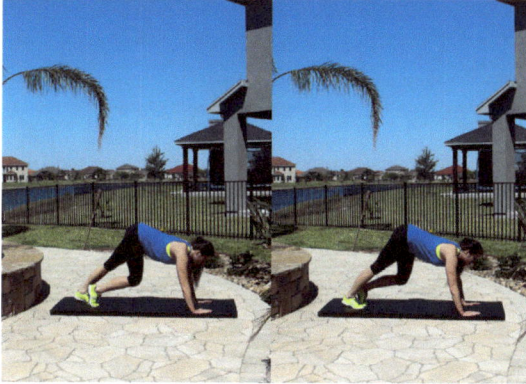

Runners Stretch

Step the left leg back into a deep lunge, placing your fingertips on the floor on either side of the right leg. Lean chest forward into the lunge until the inner thigh and groin area feel a slight stretch. Try to keep back leg fully extended.

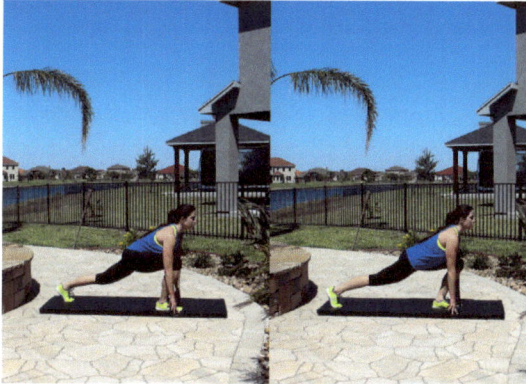

Quadriceps Stretch

Stand with feet hip width apart. Bend right knee, reaching the heal behind you and up toward the glute. Grab hold of the right foot with your right hand and stretch the right quadriceps. Then switch to the left leg.

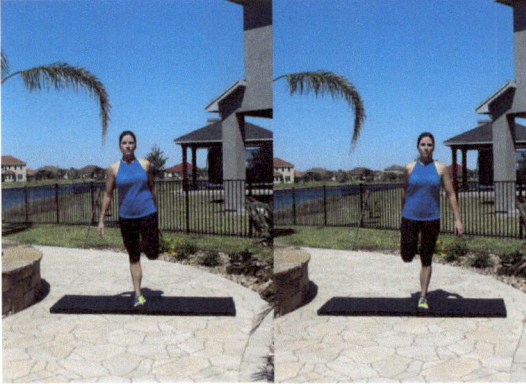

I hope you enjoyed this workout routine! Remember, as you learn new exercises, you can add them to the routine or replace other ones. Make sure to modify exercises that are not comfortable. And always consult your doctor before starting a new exercise program.

If you are making progress on your health journey, write an Amazon review for this book. I would love to hear your thoughts and read your story. Also, you can check out my other fiction and non-fiction books on Amazon that will revolutionize your heart, mind and spirit! Find me at www.alisahopewagner.com.

Blessings to your life of complete health!

alisa

www.ingramcontent.com/pod-product-compliance
Lightning Source LLC
Chambersburg PA
CBHW041303290326
41931CB00032B/11